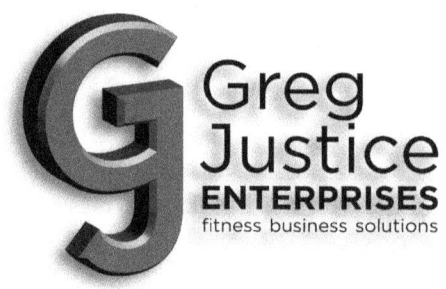

Warning:
This Material Is Copyright Protected

Published By:
GJ Enterprises
7830 State Line Rd., Ste. 101
Prairie Village, KS 66208

info@gregjustice.com

MIND OVER FATTER:
A SIX-WEEK COURSE TO A FITTER YOU!

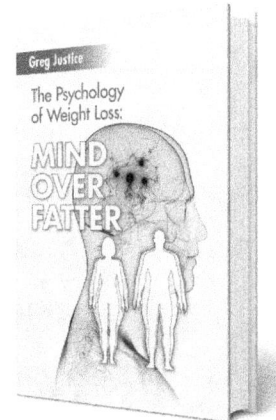

OVERVIEW

Have you thought that losing weight was something that happened to other people – and not you? Have you found yourself yo-yoing?

UPON COMPLETION OF THIS COURSE, YOU SHOULD:

1. Have the ability to recognize when you're eating to live, versus mindlessly eating due to stress or boredom.

2. Know how to deal with body dissatisfaction, and where it comes from in the first place.

3. Understand the techniques and strategies that can help you prepare for your own weight-loss journey.

4. Know how to pick the best practices and approaches to losing weight.

5. Understand how to identify the triggers that make you engage in negative eating behaviors.

6. Have the ability to keep the weight off – for life.

IN THIS COURSE, WE WILL COVER THE FOLLOWING TOPICS:

- Week One: Dealing With Your Body Dissatisfaction

- Week Two: Are You Living To Eat, Or Eating To Live?

- Week Three: Prepare For Your Journey

- Week Four: How To Set The Right Goals

- Week Five: The Lifestyle Changes You Need To Make

- Week Six: Keeping The Weight Off – For Good

INTRODUCTION

Let's face it; at some point in your life, you've tried to lose weight.

After all, you've probably picked up my *Mind Over Fatter: The Psychology of Weight Loss* – and that's what led you to this six-week course. Maybe you recognized yourself in a few of the examples I illustrated in my book. Perhaps you found yourself commiserating with feeling bad about yourself every time you eat a meal, or you recognized yourself in my description of someone who has made a habit of just mindlessly eating in front of the television.

(And if you haven't read my book, don't worry; this six-week course will be pretty self-explanatory. But do yourself a favour and pick up a copy of *Mind Over Fatter* sooner rather than later!)

No matter what truths you may have discovered in *Mind Over Fatter*, there was one thought that led you to this special six-week course:

"I'm ready to break free from the cycle of mindless, toxic, and unhealthy eating."

That's precisely where this six-week course comes into play. This course has been designed to complement *Mind Over Fatter*. Think of my book as the "big picture", with this course providing the strategies and techniques required to master emotional and mental control over weight loss.

The *Mind Over Fatter* six-week course is designed to give you highly effective – and mercifully simple – techniques that you can implement within seven days. Each week is meant to build upon one another, so by the time you reach the end, you will be practically an expert on mastering emotional and mental eating triggers.

Why six weeks? Well, evidence suggests that it takes anywhere from four to twelve weeks to learn a new habit. In terms of emotional and mental eating, six weeks can help you get in touch with the triggers that set off your eating, along with what's holding you back from actually losing the weight. Remember, this isn't a traditional diet-and-exercise plan that details everything you need to put into your mouth to lose weight in time for swimsuit season.

Think of this as your appointment with an inexpensive food therapist – one who will teach you to make connections between the foods you eat, why you eat them, and what triggers are causing you to eat more than you actually need.

I'll refer back to key points in *Mind Over Fatter* throughout the duration of the course. While I'll offer brief recaps on the bigger ideas from my book, you might find it beneficial to look back to the book if you need any refreshers on big picture ideas and terms.

Ready to get started on your six-week journey to emotional and mental mastery over weight loss? Of course you are; so get out a pen and paper, mark your calendars, and get ready to transform the way you look at weight loss in just a month and a half!

WEEK ONE: DEALING WITH YOUR BODY DISSATISFACTION

Let's do a quick exercise to start this first week. During the next seven days, we're going to get down to the nitty-gritty of why you feel the way you do when you think about your body. This exercise will help us set the foundation for the next five weeks, as it can help you identify emotional and mental triggers that might undermine your weight-loss journey.

EXERCISE 1.1

Stand in front of the mirror with no clothes on (obviously, you should do this exercise when you have as much privacy as possible). Using a pen and a pad of paper, write down the good things you see about your body. Don't edit yourself; just write down the first things that come to mind.

Once you've mentioned all the positive things about your body, you know what's next – write down everything about your body that makes you feel uncomfortable, sad, or just gives you an overall negative impression. Again, don't edit or censor yourself; just write down the first things that come to mind.

Now take a look at what you've written down about your body. Which list is longer? Positive or negative?

Don't go into the minutia of what you wrote down; just quickly assess which list is longer in terms of quantity.

If you're like nine out of ten Americans, it's likely you wrote down more negative qualities about your body than positive ones. Unfortunately, we live in a society where we're constantly pushing ourselves to achieve absolute physical perfection, even in the face of "photoshopped," unrealistic expectations. Men find themselves pushing to be the strongest, most physically fit person at the gym, and women are constantly dieting themselves into starvation, always striving to achieve that magical number where all of their problems will instantly disappear.

In *Mind Over Fatter*, I mention that a recent survey by The Calorie Control Council revealed that 82% of the population is either dissatisfied with their weight, wishing to reduce their weight, or are trying to control or maintain their weight. Out of 100 million dieters, 20 million dieters average four to five attempts each year to lose weight. According to the National Eating Disorders Association, on any given day, 45% of women are on a diet, and a whopping 40% of those women would exchange three to five years of life to have their weight loss goals satisfied.

That's a LOT of energy being used up in the pursuit of weight loss – and unfortunately, many people just aren't doing it in the healthiest way possible.

But all of this information begs the question: If so many people are constantly dieting, what's with all the hang-ups and obstacles preventing people from actually losing the weight?

Many people might cite a slowing metabolism or overeating as the primary reasons they just can't seem to lose the weight – and for many of these people, they'd be partially right. But that doesn't really highlight the mental reasons why so many of us are unhappy with our bodies – and why you might have put more negative qualities on your list than positive ones.

The main problem is how we view body image – and many of us find ourselves not weighing up to some preconceived notion of what it truly means to be "fit and thin."

To help you start to align the mind-body connections (which is vital toward building a more positive body image), use the following tips and strategies:

Look Outside Of Your Body. If you focus too much on your body and how it looks, you begin to only define yourself according to your size and how you look in the mirror. That's why I want you to use this next exercise to help you realize that you're so much more than your physical appearance.

EXERCISE 1.2

Find a quiet space where you can focus and think. Grab your trusty pen and pad of paper again. Instead of writing about parts of your body that you like or dislike, I want you to write down ten things you like about yourself – *without mentioning your body.*

It's harder than it seems, isn't it? This difficulty might be due to the fact that you've been taught for so long that your value can only be found in your physical appearance, or your clothing size.

To help get you started, ask yourself the following questions:

- What do my friends say they like most about me?

- What do my family members say are my best qualities?

- Is there a skill or a talent that I'm proud of?

- What do I enjoy doing when there's no one around?

- Am I a fast learner? Persistent? Resilient?

- What do I enjoy learning about the most?

- Where have I traveled in my life?

- Where would I go if money were no object? Why?

These questions will provide a prompt for exploring what it is about you that makes you so unique, and why you're so much more than your size.

Write down the ten qualities and then do yourself a favor – stick them someplace where you'll always be able to see them. I'm talking the bathroom mirror, on your computer monitor, or even next to your bed so you can read your best qualities before you go to bed every night.

Cut Yourself Off. Listen – I know watching those reality TV shows can be addictive. I know that magazines filled with glossy pictures of impossibly fit men and women can be fun to look at. But ultimately, those pictures are like candy; they might taste good in the short-term, but they're only poisoning you over the long-term.

For the next six weeks, I challenge you to eliminate all of the negative media influences that might be present in your home. If you have fashion or fitness magazines lying around, toss them out. If you've DVR'ed every episode of your favorite reality TV program, delete it. Over the next six weeks, I'm aiming to purge as much of the toxins from your life as possible...

So, by the time you reach the six-week mark, you'll realize how much these toxic influences were holding you back from developing a truly healthy and positive relationship with your body.

Get Rid Of The Scale. You knew this was coming. If you want to start building a positive body image, you need to divorce yourself from your weight. You're worth so much more than a number on a scale – so why are you weighing (no pun intended) so much of your self-worth against it? Give your scale a break. For the next six weeks, any weight loss will be measured against how your clothes fit – and for the record, that's what you should be using to determine how much progress you've made.

After all, you could feel thinner and more confident in your clothes, only to see the numbers on the scale refuse to budge. Free your mind from the scale and watch as your body image and self-confidence soars to new levels!

Do Something Nice. Too many people are finding their self-worth based on what they and others think of their body. But looks change – your personality is forever. That's why, for the first week of the *Mind Over Fatter* course, I want you to resolve to do something genuinely nice for another person. Here are a few suggestions that can get you started:

- Volunteer at your local church this upcoming Sunday

- Give money, clothes, or food to a homeless person

- Help an older person cross the street, or reach something high up in the grocery store aisle

- Send a nice email to a friend or family member you haven't talked to in a long time

- Give an acquaintance a compliment

- Tell someone close to you that you love and appreciate them

- Spend at least an hour on your favorite hobby, or pick up a new hobby that you've always meant to try

- Eat a new cuisine you've never tried before

Notice how simple and easy these things can be? It doesn't take much to start to understand that your life – and your worth – is made up of so much more than your body. You are a person who is capable of creating beautiful experiences – none of which have to be related to your body size or type.

Stop The Negative Thoughts. I understand this is easier said than done. After all, if it were that simple to stop feeling bad about yourself, you would have done it by now. But stopping negative body talk about yourself is as simple as vocally interrupting the thought as soon as you recognize you're having it.

The next time you catch yourself in the midst of a negative thought about your body, I want you to do the following:

- Recognize the negative body thought you're having. Try to clarify it to its most simplistic form.

- Say out loud, "I know I'm having a bad thought about my body. I know that this thought isn't true."

- Tell yourself three positive things about who you are as a person. Make sure they're related to your skills, talents, and personality — not your body.

- Say those three things out loud. Repeat them as often as possible until you start to feel better about yourself (you may want to find an isolated place to do this so you don't feel embarrassed in front of other people).

Resolve to do the following activity at least once every day. It's going to take a considerable amount of self-awareness to catch your negative body talk when it happens, but that's precisely the point. You want to catch your mind whenever it dips into the negative self-talk and forcefully remind yourself of all the reasons why you're a unique and special person. Soon, you'll be able to stop negative body talk in its tracks without having to say your positive feedback out loud.

WEEK ONE: FINAL THOUGHTS

During this first week, I don't want you to put too much pressure on yourself to rigorously exercise or restrict your diet. While I'm not giving you a free pass here, I do want you to focus on a relationship you've been neglecting for some time: the one you have with your mind.

You've been using your mind to abuse your body, as well as your soul. To build the foundation for true weight-loss success — the kind where you're not yo-yo dieting for the rest of your life — you need to align your mind to more positive feedback. So take it easy on yourself, especially if you're focusing on making a more positive mind-body connection. It's perhaps the most important step you can take in putting your "mind over fatter."

WEEK TWO: ARE YOU EATING TO LIVE, OR LIVING TO EAT?

It's a scenario that is far too common.

You find yourself a few hours into your favorite television show. You begin to feel hungry, even though you ate lunch a couple of hours ago. You walk to the kitchen, grab a bag of chips, and start to mindlessly munch when you return to the couch. Before you know it, you've finished the bag of chips and there's nothing left but a cheesy crust of chip residue remaining on your fingertips.

Suddenly, you feel incredibly guilty and angry that you couldn't stop yourself from binging on the chips, even though you weren't hungry. You promise that you're never going to do it again. In fact, you might even toy with the idea of skipping your next meal to compensate for all of the extra calories.

If the above scenario sounds familiar, then it's time to acknowledge that you're caught in a cycle where you're just living to eat. This is a battle that many Americans are facing. Despite swaths of entertainment, technologies, and social media, we're feeling more bored, stressed, and emotional than ever before.

And that means we're more likely to turn to the one source of comfort we've been taught to crave since we were little – food.

In *Mind Over Fatter*, you learned what the primary differences were between emotional eating and physical eating. As a quick recap, emotional eating is the kind of eating you do when you're responding to an emotional stimulus (i.e. eating while you're bored, stressed, or sad). Physical eating stems from feeling actual hunger and using food as a way to satiate that hunger. With the latter option, someone is much more likely to stop eating as soon as the hunger goes away. With emotional eating however, people often continue eating even when they're already feeling incredibly full.

If you're not already sure, **how can you know if you're an emotional eater?** Let's take a look at a few of the biggest signs:

1. You eat even when you're not feeling hungry.

2. You find it difficult to be satisfied by food; you're always left wanting more.

3. Your cravings are triggered by emotions like anxiety, stress, or sadness rather than that tell-all rumble in your stomach.

4. There's a mindless component of your eating habits; you find yourself shocked at how much you've eaten, as you don't remember eating all of it.

If any of the above statements are true, it's highly likely you are an emotional eater. Fortunately, there are ways you can break the habit of emotional eating, and you've already set that foundation by establishing a healthier relationship between your mind and your body in the first week of this course.

Before we move onto tips and strategies to break the hold emotional eating has over you, let's take a look at some of the reasons why more people are susceptible than others to emotional eating:

- **Genetics:** Research has uncovered the FTO, or the "fatso" gene. It might sound mean, but it turns out that people with this gene are 40% more likely to be obese than those without it.

- **Belief Systems:** Remember all those times when your mom or grandma would comfort you with food after a bad day? That's precisely why many people turn to junk food when they're feeling bad about themselves. Since we were little, we've been taught that food can be a source of comfort and love.

  It's not just for negative emotions; happy occasions center on cake, ice cream, decadent meals, and overstuffing yourself (Thanksgiving, anyone?). With this in mind, it's no wonder that almost any emotion makes some people want to start snacking.

- **Convenience:** Much of emotional eating tends to center around foods that we consider to be easy and convenient. Think about it this way: When you're feeling stressed or tired, would you rather prepare a home-cooked meal or go to a vending machine or nearby fast-food joint? For most people, emotional eating comes down to finding food that's quick, easy, and convenient. Unfortunately, our society makes it all too easy for us to find.

- **Entertainment:** As I've said before, not all emotional eating involves negative emotions; happiness, excitement, and elation can all be emotions that can propel you to start snacking and drinking. Between birthday dinners, weddings, and Super Bowl parties, happy events can often involve the kind of emotional eating that's considered more "acceptable."

Now that we've moved onto the second week, we're going to start building on the basic lessons we've learned from the first week. This week, you'll learn the techniques and strategies you can start using *immediately* to help curb your emotional eating habits.

Be Aware: Emotional eating is often associated with mindless eating, simply because you're either too stressed or too bored to realize how much you're consuming. If you want to cut down your emotional eating, the best thing to do is to simply take a step back and make note of the emotions you're feeling while you're eating.

Ask yourself the following questions:

- Do I genuinely feel hungry right now?

- Do I feel full? Do I feel uncomfortably full?

- Am I eating because I'm bored or doing a mindless activity?

- Am I eating because I'm stressed out and looking for comfort?

- Am I eating something because "I deserve it" or as a reward?

Stopping the pattern of emotional eating can be extremely difficult, especially if you've been doing it for a significant amount of time. That's why it might not be enough to simply "ask" yourself these questions while you're eating. If that sounds familiar to you, then this next exercise is for you.

EXERCISE 2.1

It's time to get back in touch with your inner child – because you're about to start keeping a journal again.

Rather than writing about your latest crush or what you did that day, you're going to use this journal exclusively for writing down what you eat throughout the day, and how you felt when you were eating. The point of this journal is to be as meticulous as possible, as it may help you identify what emotions are more likely to inspire an emotional eating binge.

Whether you use a paper journal or an online diary, find a format that lets you easily record everything you eat throughout the day. List every food you've had, even if it's a handful of chips while you were cooking dinner. If you're not honest about your eating habits it will be tough to use this exercise to break the emotional eating cycle.

Once you've recorded all of the food you ate today, think back to how you felt immediately before you started to eat. Record this emotion, including how long you felt it for, and what (if any) events inspired how you felt. This process will help you identify the triggers that are likely to make you emotionally eat.

For example, if you started snacking on chips after a stressful meeting with your boss, it's likely that your emotional eating trigger was stress.

Be faithful to your journal. As the days turn into weeks, look for patterns in your emotional eating habits. For example, if you notice that lack of sleep tends to be your biggest emotional eating trigger, you'll want to take concrete steps to start getting more sleep each night.

Replace The Food: If you're feeling tempted to snack on something, replace food with something else that can help you quell the urge. Here are a few example replacements:

- If you're feeling tempted to start binging on chips, drink a glass of ice-cold water or low-calorie juice instead.

- Hold yourself off from eating for at least 15 minutes. If you're still tempted to eat after that amount of time, it's likely that you're feeling genuine hunger.

- Before reaching for those cookies, distract yourself with another activity. Start a load of laundry, call your best friend, or just start a conversation with your significant other. By the time you're done with the activity, you may discover that you're not actually hungry after all.

- Take several deep breaths before you reach for that food. Studies have shown that deep, meditative breathing can help reduce stress, which is one of the primary reasons why you might be tempted to start emotionally eating.

- Give yourself a massage. Studies have shown that when you massage your hands or your feet – or have a partner massage them for you – you're more likely to feel less stressed and anxious. Even a minute of self-massage can make you feel more relaxed, which is essential for curbing emotional eating habits.

Enlist Social Support: Connecting with others is a great way to stop yourself from emotional eating, as it creates a sense of accountability. Find someone in your life that you can trust with your mission to lose weight - someone who won't judge you for having a complicated relationship with food.

More importantly, find someone you're comfortable sharing your feelings with, especially the negative ones that may be connected to your overeating habits. Whether this is your best friend or significant other, enlisting social support can make it easier for you to rise above any emotions that are tempting you to emotionally eat.

To effectively use your social support, it's important to call up that person every time you feel tempted to start eating (this is why you might need someone who's understanding). Let them know that you're feeling the urge to emotionally eat, and have them talk you down from this feeling.

Enlisting social support can also give you a sense of responsibility and accountability, as your friend can help you keep on the straight and narrow. For example, if your friend hasn't heard from you in a couple of weeks, he or she can call you and ask you why you haven't been talking about your eating habits. This technique can ensure that you're working hard to curb your emotional eating, since you're accountable to someone.

Trick Yourself: The best way to make it harder to emotionally eat is to take the tempting snacks and foods out of your house altogether. As a rule of thumb, just assume whatever food is in your house will be eaten, even if you've told yourself that it's off limits.

EXERCISE 2.2

Ready for spring cleaning? It's time to grab a garbage bag and start cleaning out any tempting foods and snacks from your kitchen cupboards!

Take a look at all of the foods in your kitchen. Assess if these foods are genuinely healthy and nutritious, or if they're tempting snack foods. Nothing is off limits, not even your kids' snack foods. If you have a feeling that you'll end up snacking on your son's Oreos or that you'll eat several spoonfuls of that peanut butter ice cream, you'll need to toss it out.

Worried you won't be able to do it on your own? This is when you may need to enlist the aid of a supportive friend or family member. This person can be in charge of assessing whether a food is truly tempting or not. He or she can also question you if you're trying to convince yourself you won't binge on those crackers when you're feeling emotional.

Emotional eating can be a tough habit to break, but it *is* breakable. It simply involves understanding the emotional triggers that cause you to want to start mindlessly snacking. The more you know about the triggers that cause these behaviors, the more likely it is you'll be self-aware enough to understand when you're eating because you're hungry…and when you're eating to satiate a feeling.

WEEK THREE: PREPARE FOR YOUR JOURNEY

Congratulations, you've made it to Week Three!

Now that you've built a strong mental understanding of why you might have trouble losing weight, it's time to start turning this knowledge into action. Over the past two weeks, you've become more self-aware of your emotional eating triggers and why you're having trouble losing weight, as well as expert strategies you can use to start building mental strength and emotional fortitude.

Now, by taking action, I don't mean you should immediately hop on a treadmill and start severely restricting your diet (in reality, that's actually a great way to end up sabotaging your weight-loss efforts). What I mean here is that weight-loss is a journey, and like any journey, you need to prepare for the trip in order to have the best time possible.

Think about the last time you went on vacation. You probably didn't randomly decide to throw your clothes into a suitcase and head to the airport without a destination in mind. Instead, you did some research online, picked your ideal destination, and booked your hotel and airfare. You researched different activities to do, and then packed accordingly. Maybe you even bought traveler's insurance. The point here is that you prepared for your journey so it would go as smoothly as possible – and the same rule of thumb needs to apply to your weight-loss journey.

So how can you prepare for a smooth and relatively trouble-free weight-loss journey? Simple. Use the Week Three tips and strategies from this week's session to prepare for maximum weight loss!

Use Your Food Journal: By now, you've had a couple of weeks experience with using your food journal (and if you haven't been consistent, now is the time to get back into it!). Your food journal is going to hold the key to your weight-loss success. By tracking what you eat – as well as the emotions you're feeling while you're eating – you can ensure that you minimize stress triggers while understanding the kinds of foods you're consuming.

At this point, I just have this to say: Keep up the good work! Continue tracking your foods, write down the quantity of what you eat, and summarize how you felt about your meal choices at the end of the day. You may even want to use your food journal to start setting goals for what you'll eat the next day (not to worry, we'll talk about this in Week Four).

Start Off Small: Remember how I said that if you immediately dive into restricting your diet, you'll probably end up failing? That's because any massive change isn't likely to stick because it's too big of a shock to your system. This week, all I want you to do is pick something small that you're going to start doing for your exercise and dieting. That way, you're more likely to incorporate this new habit into your everyday life, and that in turn adds up to significant weight-loss success.

Pick one or two of the following options (remember, try not to do it all at once, as you might end up stressing yourself out with all of the change):

- Add a healthy portion of green vegetables to every meal.

- Add a piece of fruit to your breakfast.

- Cook a meatless meal a few times a week.

- Go for a ten-minute walk three times a day.

- Have one carb-free meal each day.

- Attend a new exercise class at a local gym once a week.

See how easy these little changes can be? If you want to keep the weight off, consistent little changes can help you adopt these habits into your everyday life. Pick a couple from the list above and resolve to use Week Three as your opportunity to try them out. Add a new change each week to the ones you're already using, as this will help you build upon your successes for significant weight loss.

Shop Smart: Grocery shopping can be a landmine of poor decisions, especially when you're just starting off on a healthier diet regimen. That's why it's important to shop smart with the following strategies:

- You've heard it before, and I'll say it here again – never go grocery shopping while you're hungry! That's a great recipe for buying everything that looks good to your hungry eyes (and stomach!). Fill up on a nutritious meal before you go grocery shopping so you can save your stomach – not to mention your wallet – from all the temptation.

- Shop around the perimeter of the aisles within the grocery store. This is where you'll find produce, meats, fresh bread, eggs, dairy, and other necessities. The middle aisles are where you'll often run into tempting foods, like cookies and chips. If you stay around the perimeter, you can fill up your cart with the food that you need to stay healthy without tempting yourself.

- This week, resolve to put more fruits and vegetables in your cart. Even if you buy frozen vegetables, you're still making an effort to get the nutrition you need.

- Go grocery shopping after you've done something good for yourself (for example, you went to the gym or you had a healthy breakfast). You're much less likely to fill your cart with bad foods if you're already on a healthy roll.

- Shop with a prepared list. Plan out the meals for the week, and *only* fill up on what you need.

Try the above strategies next time you go grocery shopping this week. These techniques can help ensure that you're filling up your grocery cart with healthy foods, rather than snack foods that will only serve to tempt you later.

Don't Skip A Meal: For the next week – and hopefully in the weeks after – resolve to not skip a meal. No matter how busy you are, always do your best to eat breakfast, lunch, and dinner. Remember, fewer meals do not equal lost weight; in fact, you'll find that quite the opposite can be true. When you skip food, your body's metabolism becomes extremely sluggish; when you finally *do* feed yourself again, your blood sugar spikes, which prompts your body to store food as fat, rather than energy.

Stock Smaller Plates: This week, resolve to eat your meals off of smaller plates. It's a neat visual trick that can help you eat less without feeling unfulfilled. Your eyes play a crucial role in how satiated you feel at dinnertime; if you see bigger portions on a massive dinner plate, you're more likely to eat that portion size. By using a smaller plate, you'll give yourself the visual cue to feel fuller with less food.

As you can see, preparing yourself for your weight-loss journey doesn't have to be complicated; it simply boils down to giving yourself the tools and strategies you need to "trick" yourself into losing weight. By stocking smaller plates in your kitchen and filling your cupboards with better food, you're making it easier to avoid tempting snacks and beginning to harness your overeating habits.

It's also important to mentally prepare yourself for the weight-loss journey ahead. This week, try out the following exercise to help put you in a more positive and productive place.

EXERCISE 3.1

If you've ever used a visualization or meditation technique before, then you know just how powerful it can be for helping you visualize and achieve your goals. Visualization can help motivate and inspire you, as it makes your goal feel that much more tangible.

In terms of weight loss, visualization can make it possible for you to feel more motivated to achieve your ultimate goal. When you provide yourself with positive visual cues as to how you'll look, feel, and act when you've lost weight, you're much more likely to stick to healthy eating and exercise.

During Week Three, make sure to use the following steps to start preparing your mind for your weight-loss journey:

- Find a quiet space where you can be alone without interruptions. If this is at home and you're worried about family interrupting, ask your significant other if you can have fifteen minutes to yourself. This way, you won't run the risk of being interrupted by your spouse or kids.

- Run either a white noise machine or relaxing music so you get into a more tranquil frame of mind.

- Start breathing in deeply through your nose for a count of seven, and out through your mouth for a count of seven. Continue repeating this pattern until you begin to feel yourself relax.

- With every breath, think of the reasons why you're losing weight. Maybe try thinking about the fact that you want to be healthier, or how great you'll look in your clothes. Maybe you want to lose weight so you can reduce your risk for certain diseases, or just feel better about yourself again. Clearly think of these reasons with every breath and visualize how you'll feel when you achieve these goals. Hold on to those feelings as long as you want, until you're ready to move onto the next reason.

- After visualizing these goals, remind yourself that you're a powerful and capable person. Think of all the successes you've had in the past. Whether you got into a great college or had a beautiful baby with your spouse, use these successes as reminders that you're capable of achieving so much – but only if you let yourself try.

Week Three is all about preparing yourself for the amazing weight-loss journey you're about to take – a journey that begins in Week Four!

WEEK FOUR: HOW TO SET THE RIGHT GOALS

Think about the last time you had to set goals to achieve what you wanted. Maybe you were working on a big project at work, or you were studying to get your degree. No matter what you were trying to do, it's likely you had to break down your big project into smaller goals so you could increase your chances of success.

Weight loss works the exact same way. Rather than thinking of your journey as a massive – and intimidating – end goal, it's important to think of it as a series of small, achievable, and realistic steps. After all, the person who resolves to achieve small, healthy changes each week is far more likely to succeed than the person whose only goal is to drop 50 pounds.

If not properly approached, weight-loss goals can be intimidating. For example, if you want to lose thirty or forty pounds – and that's the only goal you have – you're much more likely to get discouraged if you have a bad week or end up gaining some weight back after a steady loss. That's why Week Four is devoted to helping you understand how to set the *right* goals, as they can help motivate and push you forward when the going gets tough.

In *Mind Over Fatter*, I discussed the importance of S.M.A.R.T. goals, which stands for Specific, Measurable, Achievable, Realistic, and Timely. These types of goals help ensure that you're setting the best goals – ones that won't end up discouraging you before you've even started. For example, if you're trying to diet your way into size 4 jeans despite never having been a size 4 at any point in your life, you'll only end up discouraged as you keep falling way short of your goal. S.M.A.R.T. goals, on the other hand, help ensure that you stay motivated, healthy, and encouraged by your great progress.

Since we already discussed how to use S.M.A.R.T. goals in *Mind Over Fatter*, let's use Week Four as an opportunity to expand on your goal-setting techniques.

Set Weekly Goals: Instead of setting one massive goal that can only be attained months down the line, try setting a weekly goal instead. Doing this can help keep you focused on continued weight loss, while providing you with the regular motivation and inspiration you need to see your weight loss through to your final goal. Your weekly weight-loss goal should be no more than one or two pounds; anything else is unhealthy and unsustainable (the only exception is in the first couple of weeks of weight loss, when you could lose several pounds of water weight).

Set Larger Milestones: In the same vein as setting weekly goals, larger milestones can be set every one to three months, depending on your final weight-loss goal. A larger milestone should be a culmination of a few weeks of weight loss. For example, you could set a goal where you lost ten percent of your body weight in three months. Your weekly goals should be designed to help you hit this larger milestone. If you were 200 pounds, your weekly goal would be to lose one to two pounds per week, with an eventual milestone goal of losing 20 pounds (10% of body weight) within three months.

Adjust Your Goals Accordingly: In addition to setting S.M.A.R.T. goals, it's important to adjust them based on your weight-loss progress. Whether you've discovered that your weight-loss goals are too unrealistic or too easy to achieve (after all, you want to challenge yourself!), it's important to be honest with yourself about how you're progressing.

If you find that you're exceeding your larger milestone weight-loss goals, adjust it so that the goal is slightly bigger (for example, you could opt to lose 12% of your body weight rather than 10%). However, if you're continually falling short of your weekly or milestone weight-loss goals, it's important to adjust the goals so that they're slightly less difficult to achieve. Goals should leave you feeling encouraged, not discouraged; if you're not achieving them, you need to adjust each goal until they're challenging yet attainable.

Reward Yourself: Don't let goals go by without rewarding yourself! In the first few weeks of your weight-loss journey, make sure you reward yourself for achieving your weekly goals. Treat yourself to a new outfit you've always wanted, or to a healthy portion of your favorite food. After about three or four weeks of consistently achieving your weekly goal (remember, change it if you think it's too easy!), reserve these rewards for the larger milestone achievements. Make sure the rewards match the size of the achievement. For example, if you lose 10% of your body weight within three months, treat yourself to a weekend trip with your partner or go to a spa for a facial treatment.

During Week Four, identify the rewards you'll provide yourself as you start on your weight-loss journey. This way, you know what rewards you'll be going after, and you'll be excited to work hard to achieve each and every one!

Exercise 4.1

For many people, creating a visualization of your weekly, monthly, and even yearly goals can be enough to keep you on track. That's why this Week Four exercise is devoted to helping you create a Weight-Loss Calendar, which will help keep you accountable to your weight-loss goals.

You can use an actual calendar; however, we recommend using an online calendar or even a Word document to create your weight-loss timeline. If you're writing down all of your goals on a calendar, you might find it challenging to go back and make changes to each milestone if you need to adjust your weight-loss goals as you go. With an online calendar or document, however, you can simply make those changes on the computer, while still maintaining a clean and organized appearance.

When creating your calendar, mark down what you'd like to lose within the year. Remember to use the S.M.A.R.T. techniques contained in *Mind Over Fatter*, as this will help you ensure that your weight-loss goal is achievable.

Once you've identified the yearly goal, go back and set your milestone goals for every three months. Make sure that these smaller goals add up to your yearly goal (give yourself a little leeway in case you plateau for a period of time).

After setting the monthly goals, it's time to set your weekly goals. If you find that you'll need to lose more than one pound every week to achieve your monthly and yearly goals, you may want to adjust your yearly goal and start the process all over again. Weight-loss can be challenging, but it shouldn't be impossible. Give yourself some wiggle room for plateaus and holiday indulgences; after all, there will be times when you might not lose weight. If you give yourself this leeway, you can minimize the possibility that you'll get discouraged, all while ensuring that you're on track to achieving your ultimate weight-loss goal.

Remember to stick to the calendar and make changes whenever you need to. Don't be hard on yourself if you find that you need to lower your weight-loss goals based on your progress. You're still doing fantastic work – so you should be proud of yourself!

As you can see, Week Four is all about creating the organized and detailed timelines that will keep you on track toward achieving your goals. Half the battle in weight-loss involves keeping close track of your goals, as well as the progress you're making toward these goals. For example, if you find that you're not on track toward achieving your three-month goal, you can make changes to your weekly diet and exercise to achieve it, or you could adjust the goal because you were too ambitious in the first place.

Now that we've spent the past month planning for your weight-loss success, it's time to move to Week Five and start putting these plans into action.

WEEK FIVE: THE LIFESTYLE CHANGES YOU NEED TO MAKE

When it comes to weight-loss success, many people think it comes down to diet and exercise. While that's true to a certain extent, not all diets and workouts will help people lose the same amount of weight; in fact, some diets work like magic for some people, while other diets will help the pounds fly off of other groups of people. That's why Week Five is devoted to helping you identify the best approaches to weight loss, as well as the general lifestyle changes you need to make to optimize your weight-loss efforts.

No matter which diet you decide to adopt (whether it's Weight Watchers, the Mediterranean Diet, or the Zone Diet), it's important to ensure it's a diet that fits into your lifestyle. After all, it's a rule of thumb that no matter how enthusiastic you might be about your diet at first, you won't be able to turn it into a lifestyle change if it's not easy and enjoyable. Diets are temporary; keeping the weight off for good requires a lifestyle change, not a fad diet. Make sure that whatever diet you're tempted to use can be used for life. Otherwise, it's a strong possibility that you're going to gain all the weight back.

During Week Five, start identifying and incorporating the lifestyle changes you need to make to keep the weight off. Remember to add one or two strategies per week, as you don't want to run the risk of overwhelming yourself.

Drink More Water: Now that you have a few weeks of dieting under your belt, you've probably lost a fair amount of water weight. The more water you drink, the more efficient your body gets at flushing out toxins, salt, and other compounds that bloat your body and slow down your waste processing systems (it sounds gross, but healthy waste removal is essential to weight loss).

As a rule of thumb, make sure you drink at least eight eight-ounce glasses of water each day. This might seem like a lot, but a few large glasses of water throughout the day will be more than enough to meet your water challenge. To make this easier, drink a glass of cold water as soon as you wake up (it helps jumpstart your metabolism), drink a bottle of water with your lunch, and drink a glass of water at dinner. If you're going out for a walk or working out, count the water you drink to rehydrate as well.

Don't Restrict Your Diet: One of the worst mistakes people make when they're trying to lose weight is that they completely remove certain types of foods from their diets altogether. While this might last in the short-term (we're talking days here), restricted yet tempting foods will always win out over your diet. If you want to make lifestyle changes, you need to ensure that there's no food that's off-limits. If you want a piece of chocolate, have a piece of chocolate; otherwise, you're just going to binge on it later.

Let's take a minute to talk about the concept of cheat days here; it's a good idea in theory, but only if you're capable of controlling yourself. Use the six days out of your week to ensure that you're earning your cheat day, because otherwise, you're going to stagnate your weight-loss efforts. During your cheat day, try to step up whatever your workout might be. If you usually go for walks in the morning, try going for a light jog or a longer walk than usual. That way, you can ensure that your cheat day isn't too decadent.

Find A Fun Workout: Time and time again, research has shown that you're more likely to stick to an exercise regimen if you find it fun and invigorating. That's why, if you're going to make a lifestyle change, you need to find fun exercises that you'll actually want to do. Otherwise, you're likely to convince yourself not to work out simply because you don't like that specific physical activity.

During Week Five, resolve to try out a few different forms of exercise. Whether it's a new yoga or spinning class, running on the treadmill, or going to a group dance class, stretch your limits and try things you've never considered before. If you don't find a class you love during Week Five, keep this challenge up until you find a workout that you love. Once you find it, do it a few times a week in addition to cleaning up your eating habits. This can help make it easier for you to incorporate physical activity into your week, as you won't try to talk yourself out of exercising.

Make It A Family Affair: During Week Five, let your family know what changes you're going to make to your diet. This is especially important to do if you cook for the family, as you want to prepare them for cleaner foods and healthier meals. While you shouldn't force your family to "diet" with you, convincing them about the merits of eating healthy can get them on board with your efforts. After all, if the rest of the family is supportive of your new healthy eating habits, you're much more likely to turn your diet into a positive and productive lifestyle change.

Have Fun With It: Find a healthy diet that lets you have fun with the foods you're cooking. For example, Weight Watchers has tons of recipes for desserts and comfort foods that are hearty yet still healthy. Try taking a cooking class that focuses on using seasonal vegetables, or cook a new recipe that you've always found challenging. You may find a secret cooking talent that you never knew you had, simply because your diet is helping you push your boundaries.

Start Small With Exercise: By Week Five, you might have been stepping up your workouts, but if you're still new to physical activity, this is the week to start getting more physical. Don't start off too aggressively; Week Five is not the time you should start logging multiple hours on the gym treadmill.

Start small so you can build up your exercise habits (think Couch to 5K over the course of a few months). Resolve to walk the dog in the morning and after dinner, and add a ten-minute walk around the office block for those extra steps. Set a goal of taking a new workout class each week so you can experience a new physical activity. You can even use a race or a special event to give you the momentum you need to start making those crucial lifestyle changes. For example, you could sign up for a charity walk or run, or you could train for a long-distance bike ride at the end of the year. This can give you the motivation you need to start incorporating more physical activity in your life.

Buy A Fitness Tracker: Week Five is a great opportunity to buy a fitness tracker. These new devices have been everywhere lately, and for good reason – they help track the number of steps you take each day, and even set up challenges with other people in your area with the same fitness tracker brand. Some fitness trackers even come with heart rate monitors, which can help you get an accurate idea of how many calories you're burning each day. This can often be a wake-up call for people who may think they're burning more calories than they really are.

Week Five represents an excellent opportunity to start using the tools and strategies that can help you turn your weight-loss journey into a lifestyle change. From fitness trackers to fun gym classes – and everything in-between – Week Five is the chance to try out new things that could help inspire your efforts to get lean and healthy.

Now that we're done with Week Five, we're moving onto Week Six – the last week of the *Mind Over Fatter* course. No matter where you are in your weight-loss journey, whether this is the first time you've tried losing weight or the twentieth, Week Six is going to ensure you're set up with the habits that are going to last you for the rest of your life. This will mean never having to encounter the weight-loss yo-yo again, so you can focus on living your dream life.

Ready? Let's get started!

Week Six: Keeping the Weight Off – For Good!

During Week Five, we talked about the strategies and techniques that can be used to help ensure long-term and successful weight loss. But what happens after you achieve that magical number on the scale or can fit into the pant size you've always wanted to fit into? How can you ensure you never have to encounter the weight-loss yo-yo ever again?

As it turns out, maintenance can be just as challenging as weight loss itself. Fortunately, at this stage, you've just proven to yourself that you're capable of surmounting these challenges – all you have to do is use these tips and strategies to ensure that the weight stays off for life.

So how can you keep the weight off for good without feeling like you're constantly depriving yourself or that you can never have the foods you love again?

Stop Losing Weight: Once you reach your goal weight, it's time to start easing back on your diet or exercise routine, as the goal here isn't to lose more weight. If you're not the biggest fan of the gym, try cutting back by a session each week, or just incorporate a couple of "normal" foods into your diet. While you don't want to revert back to your older eating habits, you don't want to keep losing weight, especially if it's on the verge of becoming unhealthy.

If you still wish to continue losing weight – even after reaching your goal – meet with your doctor to discuss whether or not it's a good idea. Like with all things, weight loss can be taken to an unhealthy extreme. You don't want it to become an obsession, as this is just as unhealthy as letting yourself become obese. If your doctor tells you not to lose any more weight, ease back on the dieting and exercise.

Appreciate Your New Normal: There's a reason why a large majority of people gain back all the weight they've lost – it's because they view their diet as a temporary fix. Once they reach their goal weight, they just resume the same toxic eating patterns that led to the weight gain in the first place. That's why it's important to look at your new healthy lifestyle as your new normal, not a temporary adjustment to your eating and exercise habits.

There's going to come a time when you might long for your old life back – and that's completely normal. You might miss the days when you could just sit on the couch and eat a pizza, or order dinner without worrying about the fat and sugar you're consuming. Let yourself feel this way – ignoring it will only make the feeling come back stronger than ever. If you need to have a day where you indulge in your favorite foods, don't stop yourself; just make sure you get right back on track. Weight-loss maintenance is all about finding the balance between occasionally enjoying your favorite fatty foods and eating a clean and healthy diet. Remember, if you deprive yourself, you'll only end up binging on the foods you're trying to avoid.

Regularly Weigh Yourself: Once you've reached your goal weight, you'll need to be vigilant about your weight from here on out. While I'm not suggesting that you weigh yourself every day – that's a great way to start an unhealthy focus on your weight – it's a good way of tracking if you're gaining any weight. This way, a big weight gain won't discourage you.

The key here is to weigh yourself at the end of every week (be sure to do it in the morning, preferably without clothes). If you find that your weight is slowly creeping up week after week, it might be time to refresh your dieting efforts or start exercising more.

Be Vigilant About Meal Planning: One of the best ways to ensure you keep the weight off for good is to plan out your meals for the week. When you're vigilant about meal planning, you can ensure that you're always going to have clean and healthy meals around the house. If you're looking for recipe inspiration, head to Pinterest and look up healthy recipes. You'll find thousands of suggestions for delicious and clean meals that will leave you and your taste buds happy.

Like when you were losing weight, be sure to avoid going to the grocery store when you're hungry. Otherwise, you'll end up with a cart full of junk food.

Realize That You Are A Winner: By reaching your weight-loss goal, you've done something that large majorities of people have long struggled with. That's no small feat, and it's exactly why you should congratulate yourself on overcoming a significant challenge.

No matter what happens in the coming weeks or years – whether you gain some of the weight back or you give into a food temptation – always remind yourself that you're capable of achieving so much. When you incorporate regular positive affirmations into your everyday life, you'll help yourself realize that you're so much more than your weight. Better yet, you'll get into the frame of mind where you realize that you're in control of your weight, and not the other way around.

That's the heart of *Mind Over Fatter!*

Your Mind Over Fatter Worksheet

Now that you've completed this special *Mind Over Fatter* six-week supplement course, it's time to start putting what you've learned to good use.

On the following worksheet, write down your starting weight, as well as the date you're beginning your new lifestyle change. This worksheet will help you keep track of your weight over the coming weeks, as well as provide you the opportunity to make any changes to your weight-loss goals.

MIND OVER FATTER WORKSHEET

NAME: _____

DATE: _____

WEIGHT:_____lbs.

MY BMI:_____ (not sure where to find this? Ask your doctor or use the BMI calculator located at http://www.nhlbi.nih.gov/health/educational/lose_wt/BMI/bmicalc.htm.)

Remember, BMI isn't the final answer to whether or not you're at a healthy weight, but it can certainly help.

WAIST:_____inches

HIP: _____inches

THIGH:_____inches

UPPER ARM:_____inches

*　　　　*　　　　*　　　　*　　　　*

MY LONG-TERM WEIGHT-LOSS GOAL IS:

_____

_____

_____

I AM GIVING MYSELF _____ MONTHS TO ACHIEVE THIS GOAL.

I PLAN ON MAKING THE FOLLOWING CHANGES TO MY LIFESTYLE:

_____

_____

_____

I WILL MAKE THE FOLLOWING CHANGES TO MY DIET:

_____

_____

_____

_____

I WILL DESIGNATE_____AS MY WEEKLY "CHEAT" DAY.

I commit to abide by and follow the rules I have set to reach my personal goals. Today I am signing this commitment stating that I will not only start but finish my journey to optimal fitness and health.

Signature _____ Date: _____

Once you've filled out and signed your worksheet, be sure to keep track of your BMI, weight, and measurements. I've included several monthly entries for you to get started. Don't be discouraged if you don't lose a massive amount of weight or inches right away – slow and steady win the race!

FITNESS IS A JOURNEY, NOT A DESTINATION!

DATE: _____

MY WEIGHT:_____lbs.

MY BMI:_____

WAIST:_____inches

HIP: _____inches

THIGH:_____inches

UPPER ARM:_____inches

WHAT DID I DO WELL THIS MONTH?

_____

_____

_____

HOW CAN I IMPROVE?

_____

_____

_____

MONTH 2

DATE: _____

MY WEIGHT:_____lbs.

MY BMI:_____

WAIST:_____inches

HIP: _____inches

THIGH:_____inches

UPPER ARM:_____inches

WHAT DID I DO WELL THIS MONTH?

_____

_____

_____

HOW CAN I IMPROVE?

_____

_____

_____

MONTH 3

DATE: _____

MY WEIGHT:_____lbs.

MY BMI:_____

WAIST:_____inches

HIP: _____inches

THIGH:_____inches

UPPER ARM:_____inches

WHAT DID I DO WELL THIS MONTH?

_____

_____

_____

HOW CAN I IMPROVE?

_____

_____

_____

MONTH 4

DATE: _____

MY WEIGHT:_____lbs.

MY BMI:_____

WAIST:_____inches

HIP: _____inches

THIGH:_____inches

UPPER ARM:_____inches

WHAT DID I DO WELL THIS MONTH?

_____

_____

_____

HOW CAN I IMPROVE?

_____

_____

_____

MONTH 5

DATE: _____

MY WEIGHT:_____lbs.

MY BMI:_____

WAIST:_____inches

HIP: _____inches

THIGH:_____inches

UPPER ARM:_____inches

WHAT DID I DO WELL THIS MONTH?

_____

_____

_____

HOW CAN I IMPROVE?

_____

_____

_____

MONTH 6

DATE: _____

MY WEIGHT:_____lbs.

MY BMI:_____

WAIST:_____inches

HIP: _____inches

THIGH:_____inches

UPPER ARM:_____inches

WHAT DID I DO WELL THIS MONTH?

_____

_____

_____

HOW CAN I IMPROVE?

_____

_____

_____